Discover The Secret

to

LONG AND VIBRANT LIFE

with

Dash, Mediterranean And Mind Diets

: The Ultimate Guide to Healthy Aging

O'Christ O

Copyright © 2024 by O'Christ O

Table of Content

Chapter 1: Introduction

- The importance of healthy aging
- The benefits of the DASH, Mediterranean, and MIND diets
- The latest research on healthy aging

Chapter 2: The DASH Diet

- What is the DASH diet?
- How the DASH diet can help you live longer and healthier
- Tips for following the DASH diet

Chapter 3: The Mediterranean Diet

- What is the Mediterranean diet?
- How the Mediterranean diet can help you live longer and healthier
- Tips for following the Mediterranean diet

Chapter 4: The MIND Diet

- What is the MIND diet?
- How the MIND diet can help you live longer and healthier
- Tips for following the MIND diet

Chapter 5: Combining the Diets

- How to combine the DASH, Mediterranean, and MIND diets

for maximum health benefits

- Tips for following a combined diet

Chapter 6: Exercise and Healthy Aging

- The importance of exercise for healthy aging
- Tips for staying active as you age

Chapter 7: Mental Health and Healthy Aging

- The importance of mental health for healthy aging
- Tips for maintaining good mental health as you age

Chapter 8: Conclusion

- The key takeaways from the book
- Final thoughts on healthy aging

CHAPTER 1: INTRODUCTION

Are you ready to unlock the secrets of a long and colorful existence? Regain your strength and give your best every day?

Discover the secret to a long life with the DASH, Mediterranean and MIND diets and revitalize your health: The ultimate guide to healthy aging.

With the latest updates and expert recommendations, you can learn how to maintain a good lifestyle and enjoy every moment to the fullest.

Whether you want to improve your physical health, mental health, or everyday life, this book has everything you need to succeed.

Don't wait to start your journey to becoming a healthier, happier person.

Get your replica now and start living a beautiful life.

Definition

Healthy aging is the process of developing and maintaining functions that enable good health in old age.

It's about adopting physically and mentally healthy habits and behaviors to live a productive and meaningful life as you age.

It's about creating environments and opportunities for people to continue doing what's important to them throughout their lives.

The goal of healthy aging is to maintain physical and mental health, avoid disability, and remain active and independent.

Successful aging is a process based on three factors: good health, good mental and physical performance, and a positive approach to life.

According to the World Health Organization (WHO), healthy aging is not just about freedom from disease and frailty; it is about enabling everyone to be who they are, what they can do, and what they value.

It is also about having the skills to do something.

This includes an individual's ability to meet basic needs, learn, grow, make decisions, move, establish and maintain relationships, and contribute to society.

Several factors influence healthy aging, including exercise, diet, sleep, and mental health.

The National Institute on Aging (NIA) offers research-backed tips to improve your health and well-being as you age.

It also provides information about steps you can take to improve your physical and mental health, and the benefits of physical activity, healthy eating, and cognitive health.

Healthy aging is about creating environments and opportunities for people to continue doing what is important to them throughout their lives.

It means not only freedom from illness and infirmity, but also having the skills to enable everyone to act in accordance with their values.

Factors that influence healthy aging include: Examples: exercise, nutrition, sleep, mental health.

NIA offers research-backed tips on how to improve your health and well-being as you age.

The Importance of Healthy Aging As we age, it is important to take care of our physical, mental, and social health in order to continue living a fulfilling life.

Healthy aging is about making lifestyle choices that promote good health and prevent age-related decline.

Factors that influence healthy aging include genetics, exercise, diet, sleep, and mental health.

By taking care of your physical, mental, and cognitive health, you can prevent age-related declines in performance and maintain your quality of life as you age.

One of the main benefits of healthy aging is the ability to maintain independence and autonomy as we age.

By staying physically active, eating a healthy diet, and taking care of your mental health, you can reduce your risk of developing chronic diseases and disorders that can limit your ability to live independently.

This will help you maintain your quality of life and continue doing the things you love as you get older.

Another benefit of healthy aging is that it helps you stay socially connected and engaged with the world around you.

As we age, it's important to maintain social connections and participate in activities that bring us joy and fulfillment.

This will help you stay mentally healthy and emotionally resilient and reduce your risk of depression and other mental health problems.

In addition to these benefits, healthy aging can also help you save money on health care costs.

By taking care of your physical and mental health, you can reduce your risk of developing chronic diseases and disabilities that require expensive treatment and long-term care.

This can help you maintain financial independence and become less dependent on the support of others as you age.

Overall, healthy aging is critical to maintaining quality of life and independence in old age.

By making lifestyle choices that promote good health and prevent age-related decline, we can live fully and enjoy every moment to the fullest.

Benefits of the DASH, Mediterranean, and MIND diets

The DASH, Mediterranean, and MIND diets are the three most popular his diets in the world, and there's a reason for that.

Each of these diets has been shown to have numerous health benefits, including reducing the risk of chronic disease, improving cognitive function, and promoting healthy aging.

DASH Diet the DASH Diet (Dietary Approach to Stop Hypertension) is a heart-healthy eating plan that emphasizes fruits, vegetables, whole grains, lean proteins, and low-fat dairy products.

This diet aims to lower high blood pressure, a major risk factor for heart disease, stroke, and other health problems.

In addition to lowering blood pressure, the DASH diet has been shown to improve insulin sensitivity, lower cholesterol, and reduce the risk of developing type 2 diabetes.

Mediterranean Diet the Mediterranean Diet is a heart-healthy eating plan that emphasizes fruits, vegetables, whole grains, legumes, nuts, seeds, fish, and olive oil.

The Mediterranean diet is a dietary pattern that emphasizes the intake of fruits, vegetables, whole grains, legumes, nuts, fish, and olive oil1.

This diet is based on the traditional eating habits of people living in countries bordering the Mediterranean Sea and has been proven to reduce the risk of heart disease, stroke, and other chronic diseases.

In addition to reducing the risk of chronic disease, the Mediterranean diet has also been shown to improve cognitive function, reduce inflammation, and promote healthy aging.

MIND Diet the MIND (Mediterranean-DASH Intervention for Delayed Neurodegeneration) diet combines DASH and the Mediterranean diet to promote brain health and reduce the risk of cognitive decline and dementia that often occur with age.

The diet emphasizes fruits, vegetables, whole grains, lean proteins, and healthy fats, and limits red meat, butter and margarine, cheese, pastries, fried foods, and fast foods.

The MIND diet has been shown to improve cognitive function, reduce the risk of Alzheimer's disease, and promote healthy aging.

The DASH, Mediterranean, and MIND diets are three of the healthiest diets in the world and have numerous health benefits.

These diets can reduce your risk of chronic disease, improve cognitive function, and promote healthy aging.

Latest Research on Healthy Aging Healthy aging is the journey and process of maintaining physical, mental, and social health as we age.

Recent research on healthy aging shows that there are many factors that can influence our ability to age healthily, including genetic factors, lifestyle choices, and environmental factors.

Lifestyle choices that promote healthy aging include eating a healthy diet, being physically active, and taking care of your mental health.

Environmental factors such as pollution can also affect our age.

By making lifestyle choices that promote good health and prevent age-related decline, we can live fully and enjoy every moment to the fullest.

One of the most interesting areas of research in healthy aging is the role of nutrition in promoting health and preventing age-related decline.

The DASH, Mediterranean, and MIND diets are three of his most popular diets in the world and have been proven to have numerous health benefits.

These diets emphasize fruits, vegetables, whole grains, lean proteins, and healthy fats, and limit processed foods, sugar, and unhealthy fats.

These dietary habits can reduce your risk of chronic disease, improve cognitive function, and promote healthy aging.

Another area of research regarding healthy aging is the importance of exercise in maintaining health as we age.

Regular exercise has been proven to reduce the risk of chronic disease, improve cognitive function, and promote healthy aging.

Exercise reduces the risk of falls and other accidents and helps you maintain independence and autonomy as you age.

In addition to diet and exercise, the latest research on healthy aging also shows the importance of social contact and mental health.

Maintaining social connections and participating in activities that bring joy and fulfillment helps maintain mental health and emotional resilience, reducing the risk of depression and other mental health problems.

Taking care of your mental health can promote healthy aging and maintain your quality of life as you age.

Overall, the latest research on healthy aging shows that there are many factors that can influence our ability to age healthily.

By making lifestyle choices that promote good health and prevent age-related decline, we can live fully and enjoy every moment to the fullest.

CHAPTER 2: THE DASH DIET

What is the DASH Diet?

The DASH Diet (Dietary Approaches to Stop Hypertension) is a healthy diet to prevent or treat high blood pressure, also known as hypertension.

The diet is rich in fruits, vegetables, whole grains, lean proteins, low-fat dairy products, and low in saturated fat, cholesterol, and sodium.

The DASH diet is also rich in nutrients such as potassium, calcium, and magnesium, which are important for maintaining good health.

The DASH diet is based on the latest research on nutrition and hypertension and has been shown to be effective in lowering blood pressure in people with high blood pressure.

This diet is also effective in reducing the risk of other chronic diseases such as heart disease, stroke, and diabetes.

Additionally, the DASH diet has been shown to improve cognitive function and promote healthy aging.

How does the DASH diet work?

The DASH diet reduces the amount of sodium in your diet, which is a major cause of high blood pressure.

This food is rich in potassium, calcium, and magnesium, which counteract the effects of sodium on blood pressure.

The DASH diet is also rich in fiber, which helps lower cholesterol and improves heart health.

The DASH diet is flexible and easy to follow.

This diet does not require special foods or supplements and can be tailored to suit the needs of different people.

This diet emphasizes whole foods such as fruits, vegetables, whole grains, and lean proteins, and limits processed foods, sugar, and unhealthy fats.

The Advantages of the DASH diet

The DASH diet has numerous health benefits, including:

1. **Lowering Blood Pressure**: The DASH diet has been shown to be effective in lowering blood pressure in hypertensive patients. This diet is also effective in reducing the risk of other chronic diseases such as heart disease, stroke, and diabetes.

2. **Improves Heart Health**: The DASH diet is rich in nutrients such as potassium, calcium, and magnesium, which are important for maintaining heart health. It's also rich in fiber, which lowers cholesterol and improves heart health.

3. **Improves cognitive function**: The DASH diet has been shown to improve cognitive function and reduce the risk of cognitive decline in older adults.

4. **Promote healthy aging**: The DASH diet is rich in nutrients important for healthy aging, including potassium, calcium, and magnesium.

Their diets are also low in unhealthy fats and processed foods, which can lead to chronic disease and other health problems.

• How the DASH Diet Can Help You Live a Healthier Longer Life

The DASH Diet (Dietary Approach to Stop Hypertension) is a healthy eating plan that can help you live a healthier longer life.

This diet aims to lower high blood pressure, a major risk factor for heart disease, stroke, and other health problems.

The DASH diet is rich in fruits, vegetables, whole grains, lean proteins, low-fat dairy products, and low in saturated fat, cholesterol, and sodium.

It is also rich in nutrients important for maintaining health, such as potassium, calcium, and magnesium.

By following the DASH diet, you can reduce your risk of chronic disease, improve cognitive function, and promote healthy aging.

The DASH diet is flexible, easy to follow, and can be tailored to suit the needs of different people.

By choosing a lifestyle that promotes good health and prevents the decline of age, you can live a fulfilling life and enjoy every moment to the fullest.

 The DASH Diet is a healthy eating plan that helps you live a longer, healthier life.

This diet aims to lower high blood pressure, a major risk factor for heart disease, stroke, and other health problems.

The DASH diet is rich in fruits, vegetables, whole grains, lean proteins, low-fat dairy products, and low in saturated fat, cholesterol, and sodium.

The diet is also rich in nutrients important for maintaining good health, such as potassium, calcium, and magnesium.

 The DASH diet reduces the amount of sodium in your diet, which is a major cause of high blood pressure.

This food is rich in potassium, calcium, and magnesium, which counteract the effects of sodium on blood pressure.

The DASH diet is also rich in fiber, which helps lower cholesterol and improves heart health.

• Tips for Sticking to the DASH Diet

The DASH Diet is flexible and easy to stick to.

1. **Eat more fruits and vegetables**: Aim to consume at least 4 to 5 servings of fruits and vegetables per day.

2. **Choose whole grains:** Instead of refined grains, choose whole grains such as brown rice, quinoa, and whole wheat bread.

3. **Eat Lean Protein**: Instead of red meat, choose lean proteins like chicken, fish, and beans.

4. **Limit Sodium**: Limit sodium intake to less than 2,300 milligrams per day.

5. **Limit unhealthy fats**: Limit your intake of unhealthy fats, such as saturated fats and Tran's fats.

6. **Limit Sugar**: Limit your intake of sugar and sugary drinks.

CHAPTER 3: MEDITERRANEAN DIET

The Mediterranean Diet is a healthy eating plan inspired by the traditional eating habits of the peoples of countries bordering the Mediterranean Sea.

This diet emphasizes minimally processed, whole foods such as fruits, vegetables, whole grains, legumes, nuts, seeds, fish, and olive oil, as well as lean meats, butter and margarine, cheese, pastries, and fried foods.

The Mediterranean diet is not a strict or restrictive diet, but rather one that emphasizes fresh, whole foods and moderate amounts of red wine.

The Mediterranean diet has been shown to have numerous health benefits, including reduced risk of heart disease, stroke, and other chronic diseases.

Meals are rich in nutrients important to maintaining good health, including fiber, vitamins, minerals, and healthy fats.

The Mediterranean diet is also rich in antioxidants, which protect the body from free radical damage.

The Mediterranean diet is associated with a lower risk of heart disease, stroke, type 2 diabetes, and certain cancers.

It has also been shown to improve cognitive function and reduce the risk of Alzheimer's disease.

A recent study found that a Mediterranean diet may reduce the risk of cognitive decline2.

Another study found that a Mediterranean diet may help reduce the risk of death from cancer.

These results suggest that the Mediterranean diet may be a promising approach to maintaining overall health.

One of the main benefits of the Mediterranean diet is that it can reduce the risk of heart disease.

The diet is rich in healthy fats, such as monounsaturated and polyunsaturated fats, which lower cholesterol and reduce the risk of heart disease.

The Mediterranean diet is also rich in omega-3 fatty acids, which are important for heart health.

In addition to reducing the risk of heart disease, the Mediterranean diet has also been shown to have other health benefits.

This diet is thought to be associated with a lower risk of cancer, Alzheimer's disease, Parkinson's disease, and other chronic diseases.

The Mediterranean diet has also been shown to improve cognitive function, reduce inflammation, and promote healthy aging.

• How the Mediterranean Diet Can Help You Live Healthier and Longer

The Mediterranean Diet is a diet that focuses on whole, minimally processed foods such as fruits, vegetables, whole grains, legumes, nuts, seeds, fish, and olive oil. Also limit red meat, butter and margarine, cheese, pastries, fried foods and fast foods.

Meals are rich in nutrients important to maintaining good health, including fiber, vitamins, minerals, and healthy fats.

The Mediterranean diet has been shown to have numerous health benefits, including reduced risk of heart disease, stroke, and other chronic diseases.

This diet is also rich in antioxidants that help protect your body from free radical damage.

Following a Mediterranean diet can reduce your risk of chronic disease, improve cognitive function, and promote healthy aging.

The Mediterranean diet is easy to follow and adaptable to the needs of different people.

By choosing a lifestyle that promotes good health and prevents the decline of age, you can live a fulfilling life and enjoy every moment to the fullest.

• Tips for practicing the Mediterranean diet

The Mediterranean diet is easy to follow and adaptable to the needs of different people.

Here are some tips for practicing the Mediterranean diet:

1. **Eat more fruits and vegetables**: Try to eat at least 4 to 5 servings of fruits and vegetables a day.

2. **Choose whole grains**: Instead of refined grains, choose whole grains such as brown rice, quinoa, and whole wheat bread.

3. **Eat Lean Protein**: Instead of red meat, choose lean proteins like chicken, fish, and beans.

4. **Use healthy fats:** Use healthy fats like olive oil, nuts, and seeds instead of butter or margarine.

5. **Limit your red meat intake**: Limit your red meat intake to a few times a month.

6. **Drink red wine in moderation**: If you drink alcohol, limit it to one drink per day for women and two drinks per day for men.

 The Mediterranean diet is a healthy eating plan that can help reduce your risk of chronic disease and improve your overall health.

CHAPTER 4: MIND DIET

• What is the MIND Diet?

MIND (Mediterranean-DASH Intervention for Neurodegenerative Delay) diet therapy protects brain function and prevents age-related cognitive decline and cognition.

A healthy eating plan that aims to prevent neurodegeneration such as neurodegeneration.

The Mediterranean Diet is based on the eating habits of people living in Mediterranean countries and has been shown to improve cardiovascular health.

Another is the DASH meal plan created by National Heart, Lung and Blood Institute is designed to lower blood pressure and improve heart health.

The MIND diet combines elements of two other plans with the goal of reducing the risk of cognitive decline and dementia that often occurs with age. It is flexible and easy to follow.

This diet emphasizes minimally processed, whole foods such as fruits, vegetables, whole grains, legumes, nuts, seeds, fish, and olive oil, as well as lean meats, butter and margarine, cheese, pastries, and fried foods.

The MIND diet is also rich in nutrients important for good health, including fiber, vitamins, minerals, and healthy fats. By following this Diet, you can reduce your risk of chronic disease, improve cognitive function, and promote healthy aging.

The MIND Diet is a scientifically proven nutritional plan designed to protect brain function and prevent age-related neurodegeneration such as cognitive decline and dementia.

The Mediterranean diet is based on the eating habits of people living in Mediterranean countries and has been shown to improve cardiovascular health.

The DASH meal plan was developed by the National Heart, Lung, and Blood Institute to lower blood pressure and improves heart health.

The MIND diet combines elements of two other plans with the goal of reducing the risk of cognitive decline and dementia that often occurs with age.

The MIND diet is flexible and easy to follow.

This diet emphasizes minimally processed, whole foods such as fruits, vegetables, whole grains, legumes, nuts, seeds, fish, and olive oil, as well as lean meats, butter and margarine, cheese, pastries, and fried foods.

The MIND diet is also rich in nutrients important for good health, including fiber, vitamins, minerals, and healthy fats.

The MIND Diet is based on the latest research in nutrition and cognitive health. This diet has been shown to have many health benefits, including reducing the risk of cognitive decline and dementia.

The MIND diet is also effective in reducing the risk of chronic diseases such as heart disease, stroke, and diabetes.

Additionally, the MIND diet has been shown to improve cognitive function and promote healthy aging.

· How the MIND Diet Can Help You Live a Longer, Healthier Life

The MIND Diet is a Scientifically Proven Diet Designed to Protect Brain Function and Reduce the Risk of Alzheimer's Disease nutrition plan.

It is a combination of the Mediterranean diet and the DASH diet, both known for their health benefits.

The MIND diet focuses on eating foods rich in nutrients such as vitamins, minerals, and antioxidants.

These foods include leafy greens, berries, nuts, whole grains, fish, and poultry.

It also recommends limiting your intake of unhealthy foods such as red meat, butter, cheese, and fried foods.

Recent observations show that the Mind Diet is associated with improved overall cognitive performance, even in older adults. This study found that consuming up to 53% of the MIND diet program can reduce the risk of cognitive decline and dementia.

Another study found that following the MIND diet increased life expectancy for women and men by more than 10 years. Additionally, the MIND diet is associated with a lower risk of depression and anxiety.

It has also been linked to a lower risk of heart disease, stroke, and type 2 diabetes.

In summary, it helps people live longer, healthier lives by protecting brain function and reducing the risk of Alzheimer's disease.

Eating nutrient-dense foods and limiting unhealthy foods can improve cognitive performance and reduce the risk of cognitive decline and dementia.

• Tips for Sticking to the MIND Diet

The MIND Diet is easy to follow and can be customized to suit the needs of different people.

Here are some tips for following the MIND diet:

1. **Eat more fruits and vegetables:** Try to eat at least 4 to 5 servings of fruits and vegetables per day.

2. **Choose whole grains**: Instead of refined grains, choose whole grains such as brown rice, quinoa, and whole wheat bread.

3. **Eat lean proteins**: Instead of red meat, choose lean proteins such as chicken, fish, and beans.

4. **Use healthy fats**: Use healthy fats like olive oil, nuts, and seeds instead of butter or margarine.

5. **Limit Red Meat**: Limit your red meat intake to a few times a month.

6. **Limit unhealthy fats**: Limit your intake of unhealthy fats, such as saturated fats and Tran's fats.

7. **Limit Sugar**: Limit your intake of sugar and sugary drinks.

Recommended fruits on the MIND diet:

• **Berries**: Berries, such as strawberries, blueberries, raspberries, and blackberries, are rich in antioxidants and are associated with improved brain function.

• **Other Fruits**: The MIND diet generally does not emphasize eating fruit, but it does encourage eating lots of fruit.

Eating fruit is associated with improved brain function, and berries in particular are supported by the strongest evidence.

Recommended vegetables for the MIND diet:

• **Green leafy vegetables** such as kale, spinach, cooked vegetables, and salads.

• **All other vegetables**: In addition to green leafy vegetables, try to eat another vegetable at least once a day.

It is best to choose non-starchy vegetables, as they provide many nutrients with low calories.

Whole grains recommended in the MIND diet:

- **Oatmeal**: Oatmeal is an excellent source of fiber and helps lower bad cholesterol levels.

It contains antioxidants, which helps to reduce inflammation.

- **Quinoa**: Quinoa is an excellent source of protein and fiber.

It contains vitamins and minerals such as magnesium, potassium, and iron.

- **Brown rice**: Brown rice is an excellent source of fiber and helps lower bad cholesterol levels.

It is also rich in vitamins and minerals such as magnesium and selenium.

- **Whole Wheat Pasta**: Whole Wheat Pasta is an excellent source of fiber and helps lower cholesterol.

It contains vitamins and minerals such as iron and zinc.

- **100% Whole Wheat Bread**: 100% Whole Wheat Bread is a good source of fiber and helps lower bad cholesterol.

It is also rich in vitamins and minerals such as magnesium and selenium

Lean protein sources recommended in the MIND diet:

- **White fish** such as cod, haddock, grouper, halibut, tilapia, and sea bass. These fish are very lean, with less than 3 g of fat, 20-25 g of protein, and 85-130 calories per 100 g cooked.

- **Greek yogurt** is an excellent source of protein. A 100g serving of regular yogurt contains about 9g of protein, compared to only about 4g.

- **Legumes** such as lentils and beans are a good source of plant protein. It's low in fat and high in fiber, making it a healthy addition to your diet.

- **Low-fat cottage cheese** is an excellent source of protein. Contains approximately 11g of protein per 100g.

• **Tofu** is an excellent source of vegetable protein. Contains approximately 8g of protein per 100g.

Healthy fats promoted in the MIND diet:

• **Avocados**: Avocados are a good source of monounsaturated fats, which lower bad cholesterol and reduce the risk of heart disease.

It is also rich in vitamin E, which fights free radical damage and boosts immunity.

• **Fatty Fish**: Fatty fish such as salmon, herring, and mackerel are rich in omega-3 fatty acids, which help reduce inflammation and lower the risk of heart disease.

• **Nuts and Seeds**: Almonds, walnuts, chia seeds, and flaxseeds, are rich in healthy fats, fiber, and protein. These can help reduce inflammation, lower bad cholesterol, and improve heart health.

• **Olive Oil**: Olive oil is a good source of monounsaturated fats and antioxidants, which can help reduce inflammation and lower your risk of heart disease.

• **Coconut Oil**: Coconut oil is an excellent source of medium chain triglycerides (MCTs) that boost metabolism and promote weight loss. It is also rich in lauric acid, which has antibacterial properties.

Here are some example meal plans to help guide you.

1: **Breakfast**

• Walnut and Blueberry Oatmeal

• Whole Wheat Toast with Almond Butter

• Coffee or Tea Lunch

• Grilled Salmon with Mixed Vegetables and Olive Oil Dressing

• Whole Wheat Roll

- Apple Dinner
- Fried Chicken with Vegetables and Brown Rice
- Glass of Red Wine Snack
- Handful of Almonds

Diet - Meal Plan

• Breakfast:

Greek Yogurt with Berries and Walnuts

• Snack: Apple Slices with Almond Butter

Lunch:

Grilled Chicken Salad with Vegetables, Tomato, Cucumber and Avocado

Snack:

Carrot and Hummus

Dinner:

Baked Salmon with Roasted Asparagus and Quinoa

Snack:

Dark Chocolate

MIND Diet Shopping List

• Fresh fruits: Berries, apples, bananas, oranges, etc.

• Fresh vegetables: Leafy vegetables, carrots, cucumbers, tomatoes, asparagus, etc.

• Nuts: Walnuts, almonds, cashews, etc.

• Seeds: Pumpkin seeds, sunflower seeds, etc.

• Legumes: Chickpeas, lentils, beans, etc.

• Whole grains: Quinoa, brown rice, whole grain bread, etc.

- Lean protein: Chicken, turkey, fish, etc.

- Healthy fats: Olive oil, avocado, etc.

- Dark chocolate

Here are some recipes for breakfast, lunch, and dinner.

Breakfast

1. **Mediterranean Omelette**: Mix 2 eggs with 1 tablespoon milk. Add 1/4 cup chopped tomatoes, 1/4 cup chopped spinach, 1/4 cup chopped mushrooms, and 1/4 cup crumbled feta cheese. Cook in a non-stick pot over medium heat until set.

2. **Blueberry Almond Smoothie**: Blend 1 cup unsweetened almond milk, 1/2 cup frozen blueberries, 1/2 banana, 1 tablespoon almond butter, and 1/2 teaspoon honey until smooth.

3. **Greek Yogurt Parfait**: Combine 1 cup plain Greek yogurt, 1/2 cup mixed berries, and 1/4 cup granola in a glass.

Lunch

1. **Mediterranean Salad**: Combine 2 cups mixed vegetables, 1/2 cup cherry tomatoes, 1/4 cup cucumber slices, 1/4 cup red onion slices, and 1/4 cup crumbled feta cheese. 1/4 cup Kalamata olives. Coat with olive oil and lemon juice.

2. **Salmon Quinoa Bowl**: Cook 1/2 cup quinoa according to package directions. Top with 4 ounces of grilled salmon, 1/4 cup sliced avocado, 1/4 cup sliced cucumber, and 1/4 cup sliced red onion. Coat with olive oil and lemon juice.

3. **Turkey Hummus Wrap**: Spread 2 tablespoons of hummus on whole wheat wrap.

Top with 2 turkey breast slices, 1/4 cup cucumber slices, 1/4 cup red onion slices, and 1/4 cup mixed vegetables. Roll it up and cut it in half.

Dinner

1. **Mediterranean Chicken**: Season 4 Add 1 teaspoon dried oregano, 1/2 teaspoon garlic powder, and 1/4 teaspoon salt to the chicken breasts. Grill until everything is cooked through. Serve with 1/2 cup cooked quinoa and 1 cup roasted vegetables.

2. **Salmon and Asparagus**: Preheat oven to 400°F. Place 4 salmon fillets and 1 bunch of asparagus on a baking sheet. Coat with olive oil and sprinkle with salt and pepper. Bake for 12 to 15 minutes, until salmon is cooked through and asparagus is tender.

3. **Mediterranean stuffed peppers**: Cut off the tops of 4 peppers and remove the seeds. In a bowl, combine 1 pound ground turkey, 1/2 cup cooked quinoa, 1/4 cup chopped Kalamata olives, 1/4 cup crumbled feta cheese, 1/4 cup chopped parsley, and 1/2 teaspoon dried oregano. Use 2 teaspoons of garlic powder and 1/4 teaspoon of salt. Stuff the peppers with the turkey mixture. Bake at 180C for 30-35 minutes, until the peppers are soft and the filling is cooked through.

Breakfast

1. **Mediterranean Breakfast Bowl**: Cook 1/2 cup quinoa according to package directions. Top with 1/4 cup hummus, 1/4 cup chopped tomatoes, 1/4 cup chopped cucumber, 1/4 cup crumbled feta cheese, and 1/4 cup Kalamata olives.

2. **Chia Seed Pudding**: Combine 1/4 cup chia seeds, 1 cup unsweetened almond milk, 1 tablespoon honey, and 1/2 teaspoon vanilla extract. Refrigerate overnight. Top with fresh berries.

3. **Mediterranean Frittata**: Mix 4 eggs with 1/4 cup milk. Add 1/4 cup chopped tomatoes, 1/4 cup chopped spinach, 1/4 cup chopped mushrooms, and 1/4 cup crumbled feta cheese. Cook in a non-stick pot over medium heat until set.

Lunch

1. **Mediterranean Wrap**: Spread 2 tablespoons of hummus on whole wheat wrap. Top with 1/4 cup mixed vegetables, 1/4 cup

chopped tomatoes, 1/4 cup chopped cucumber, 1/4 cup sliced red onion, 1/4 cup crumbled feta cheese, and 1/4 cup Kalamata olives. Roll it up and cut it in half.

2. **Salmon Salad**: Combine 2 cups mixed vegetables, 4 ounces grilled salmon, 1/4 cup sliced avocado, 1/4 cup sliced cucumber, and 1/4 cup sliced red onion. Coat with olive oil and lemon juice.

3. **Mediterranean Tuna Salad**: 1 can drained tuna, 1/4 cup chopped Kalamata olives, 1/4 cup chopped red onion, 1/4 cup chopped cucumber, 1/4 cup chopped tomatoes, and 1/4 cup crushed. Coat with olive oil and lemon juice.

Dinner

1. **Mediterranean Grilled Chicken**: Season chicken breasts with 1 teaspoon dried oregano, 1/2 teaspoon garlic powder, and 1/4 teaspoon salt. Grill until everything is cooked through. Serve with 1/2 cup cooked quinoa and 1 cup roasted vegetables.

2. **Salmon and Sweet Potatoes**: Preheat oven to 400°F. Place 4 salmon fillets and 2 sweet potatoes on a baking sheet. Coat with olive oil and sprinkle with salt and pepper. Bake for 12 to 15 minutes, until the salmon is cooked through and the sweet potatoes are tender.

3. **Mediterranean Stuffed Zucchini**: Cut 4 zucchini in half lengthwise and scoop out seeds. In a bowl, combine 1 pound ground turkey, 1/2 cup cooked quinoa, 1/4 cup chopped Kalamata olives, 1/4 cup crumbled feta cheese, 1/4 cup chopped parsley, and 1/2 teaspoon dried oregano. Use 2 teaspoons of garlic powder and 1/4 teaspoon of salt. Stuff the zucchini with the turkey mixture. Bake at 180°C for 30-35 minutes, until the zucchini is soft and the inside is cooked through.

Day 1

• **Breakfast:**

Mediterranean omelette. Whisk 2 eggs with 1 tablespoon of milk.

Add 1/4 cup chopped tomatoes, 1/4 cup chopped spinach, 1/4 cup chopped mushrooms, and 1/4 cup crumbled feta cheese. Cook in a non-stick pot over medium heat until set.

· Lunch:

Mediterranean Salad. Combine 2 cups mixed vegetables, 1/2 cup cherry tomatoes, 1/4 cup cucumber slices, 1/4 cup red onion slices, 1/4 cup crumbled feta cheese, and 1/4 cup Kalamata olives. Coat with olive oil and lemon juice.

· Dinner:

Mediterranean Chicken. Season the chicken breast from step 4 with 1 teaspoon dried oregano, 1/2 teaspoon garlic powders, and 1/4 teaspoon salt. Grill until everything is cooked through. Serve with 1/2 cup cooked quinoa and 1 cup roasted vegetables.

Day 2

· Breakfast:

Mediterranean Breakfast Bowl. Follow the package instructions to cook 1/2 cup of quinoa. Top with 1/4 cup hummus, 1/4 cup chopped tomatoes, 1/4 cup chopped cucumber, 1/4 cup crumbled feta cheese, and 1/4 cup Kalamata olives.

· Lunch:

Salmon salad. Combine 2 cups mixed vegetables, 4 ounces grilled salmon, 1/4 cup sliced avocado, 1/4 cup sliced cucumber, and 1/4 cup sliced red onion. Coat with olive oil and lemon juice.

· Dinner:

 Salmon and sweet potato. Preheat oven to 400°F. Place 4 salmon fillets and 2 sweet potatoes on a baking sheet. Coat with olive oil and sprinkle with salt and pepper. Bake for 12-15 minutes until the salmon is cooked through and the sweet potatoes are tender.

Day 3

• **Breakfast**: Chia Seed Pudding. Mix 1/4 cup chia seeds, 1 cup unsweetened almond milk, 1 tablespoon honey, and 1/2 teaspoon vanilla extract. Refrigerate overnight. Top with fresh berries.

• **Lunch**:

Mediterranean Tuna Salad. 1 can drained tuna, 1/4 cup chopped kalamata olives, 1/4 cup chopped red onion, 1/4 cup chopped cucumber, 1/4 cup chopped tomatoes, 1/4 cup crumbled feta cheese. Coat with olive oil and lemon juice.

• **Dinner**:

Mediterranean Stuffed Zucchini. Cut 4 zucchini in half lengthwise and scoop out the seeds. In a bowl, combine 1 pound ground turkey, 1/2 cup cooked quinoa, 1/4 cup chopped Kalamata olives, 1/4 cup crumbled feta cheese, 1/4 cup chopped parsley, and 1/2 teaspoon dried oregano. Use 2 teaspoons of garlic powder and 1/4 teaspoon of salt. Stuff the zucchini with the turkey mixture. Bake at 180°C for 30-35 minutes, until the zucchini is soft and the inside is cooked through.

Day 4

• **Breakfast**: Greek yogurt parfait. Combine 1 cup plain Greek yogurt, 1/2 cup mixed berries, and 1/4 cup granola in a glass.

• **Lunch**:

Mediterranean Wrap. Spread 2 tablespoons of hummus on whole wheat wrap. Top with 1/4 cup mixed vegetables, 1/4 cup chopped tomatoes, 1/4 cup chopped cucumber, 1/4 cup sliced red onion, 1/4 cup crumbled feta cheese, and 1/4 cup Kalamata olives. Roll it up and cut it in half.

• **Dinner**:

Mediterranean grilled chicken. Season the chicken breast from step 4 with 1 teaspoon dried oregano, 1/2 teaspoon garlic powders, and 1/4 teaspoon salt. Grill until everything is cooked through. Serve with 1/2 cup cooked quinoa and 1 cup roasted vegetables.

Day 5

· **Breakfast:**

Mediterranean Frittata. Whisk 4 eggs with 1/4 cup milk. Add 1/4 cup chopped tomatoes, 1/4 cup chopped spinach, 1/4 cup chopped mushrooms, and 1/4 cup crumbled feta cheese. Cook in a non-stick pot over medium heat until set.

· **Lunch:**

Salmon Quinoa Bowl. Cook 1/2 cup quinoa according to package directions. Top with 4 ounces of grilled salmon, 1/4 cup sliced avocado, 1/4 cup sliced cucumber, and 1/4 cup sliced red onion. Coat with olive oil and lemon juice.

· **Dinner:**

Salmon and asparagus. Preheat oven to 400°F. Place 4 salmon fillets and 1 bunch of asparagus on a baking sheet. Coat with olive oil and sprinkle with salt and pepper. Bake for 12 to 15 minutes, until salmon is cooked through and asparagus is tender.

Day 6

· **Breakfast:**

Blueberry Almond Smoothie. Mix 1 cup unsweetened almond milk, 1/2 cup frozen blueberries, 1/2 banana, 1 tablespoon almond butter, and 1/2 teaspoon honey until smooth.

· **Lunch:**

Turkey Hummus Wrap. Spread 2 tablespoons of hummus on whole wheat wrap. Top with 2 turkey breast slices, 1/4 cup cucumber slices, 1/4 cup red onion slices, and 1/4 cup mixed vegetables. Roll it up and cut it in half.

· **Dinner:**

Mediterranean stuffed peppers with meat. Cut off the tops of 4 peppers and remove the seeds. In a bowl, combine 1 pound ground turkey, 1/2 cup cooked quinoa, 1/4 cup chopped

Kalamata olives, 1/4 cup crumbled feta cheese, 1/4 cup chopped parsley, and 1/2 teaspoon dried oregano. Use 2 teaspoons of garlic powder and 1/4 teaspoon of salt. Stuff the peppers with the turkey mixture. Bake at 180C for 30-35 minutes, until the peppers are soft and the filling is cooked through.

Day 7

· **Breakfast**:

Mediterranean Breakfast Bowl. Follow the package instructions to cook 1/2 cup of quinoa. Top with 1/4 cup hummus, 1/4 cup chopped tomatoes, 1/4 cup chopped cucumber, 1/4 cup crumbled feta cheese, and 1/4 cup Kalamata olives.

· **Lunch**:

Mediterranean Tuna Salad. 1 can drained tuna, 1/4 cup chopped kalamata olives, 1/4 cup chopped red onion, 1/4 cup chopped cucumber, 1/4 cup chopped tomatoes, 1/4 cup crumbled feta cheese. Drizzle with olive oil and lemon juice.

· **Dinner**:

Mediterranean grilled chicken. Season the chicken breast from step 4 with 1 teaspoon dried oregano, 1/2 teaspoon garlic powders, and 1/4 teaspoon salt. Grill until everything is cooked through. Serve with 1/2 cup cooked quinoa and 1 cup roasted vegetables.

Day 8

· **Breakfast**:

Chia seed pudding. Mix 1/4 cup chia seeds, 1 cup unsweetened almond milk, 1 tablespoon honey, and 1/2 teaspoon vanilla extract. Refrigerate overnight. Top with fresh berries.

· **Lunch**:

Mediterranean Wrap. Spread 2 tablespoons of hummus on whole wheat wrap. Top with 1/4 cup mixed vegetables, 1/4 cup chopped tomatoes, 1/4 cup chopped cucumber, 1/4 cup sliced red onion, 1/4 cup crumbled feta cheese, and 1/4 cup Kalamata olives. Roll it up and cut it in half.

· Dinner:

Mediterranean Stuffed Zucchini. Cut 4 zucchini in half lengthwise and scoop out the seeds. In a bowl, combine 1 pound ground turkey, 1/2 cup cooked quinoa, 1/4 cup chopped Kalamata olives, 1/4 cup crumbled feta cheese, 1/4 cup chopped parsley, and 1/2 teaspoon dried oregano. Use 2 teaspoons of garlic powder and 1/4 teaspoon of salt. Stuff the zucchini with the turkey mixture. Bake at 180°C for 30-35 minutes, until the zucchini is soft and the inside is cooked through.

Day 9

· Breakfast:

Greek yogurt parfait. Combine 1 cup plain Greek yogurt, 1/2 cup mixed berries, and 1/4 cup granola in a glass.

· Lunch:

Salmon Quinoa Bowl. Follow the package instructions to cook 1/2 cup of quinoa. Top with 4 ounces of grilled salmon, 1/4 cup sliced avocado, 1/4 cup sliced cucumber, and 1/4 cup sliced red onion. Drizzle with olive oil and lemon juice.

· Dinner:

Salmon and asparagus. Preheat oven to 400°F. Place 4 salmon fillets and 1 bunch of asparagus on a baking sheet. Coat with olive oil and sprinkle with salt and pepper. Bake for 12 to 15 minutes, until salmon is cooked through and asparagus is tender.

Day 10

· Breakfast:

Blueberry Almond Smoothie. Mix 1 cup unsweetened almond milk, 1/2 cup frozen blueberries, 1/2 banana, 1 tablespoon almond butter, and 1/2 teaspoon honey until smooth.

- **Lunch:**

Turkey Hummus Wrap. Spread 2 tablespoons of hummus on whole wheat wrap. Top with 2 turkey breast slices, 1/4 cup cucumber slices, 1/4 cup red onion slices, and 1/4 cup mixed vegetables. Roll it up and cut it in half.

- **Dinner:**

Mediterranean stuffed peppers with meat. Cut off the tops of 4 peppers and remove the seeds. In a bowl, combine 1 pound ground turkey, 1/2 cup cooked quinoa, 1/4 cup chopped Kalamata olives, 1/4 cup crumbled feta cheese, 1/4 cup chopped parsley, and 1/2 teaspoon dried oregano. Use 2 teaspoons of garlic powder and 1/4 teaspoon of salt. Stuff the peppers with the turkey mixture. Bake at 180C for 30-35 minutes, until the peppers are soft and the filling is cooked through.

Day 11

- **Breakfast:**

Mediterranean Breakfast Bowl. Cook 1/2 cup quinoa according to package directions. Top with 1/4 cup hummus, 1/4 cup chopped tomatoes, 1/4 cup chopped cucumber, 1/4 cup crumbled feta cheese, and 1/4 cup Kalamata olives.

- **Lunch:**

Mediterranean Tuna Salad. 1 can drained tuna, 1/4 cup chopped kalamata olives, 1/4 cup chopped red onion, 1/4 cup chopped cucumber, 1/4 cup chopped tomatoes, 1/4 cup crumbled feta cheese. Coat with olive oil and lemon juice.

- **Dinner:**

Mediterranean grilled chicken. Season the chicken breast from step 4 with 1 teaspoon dried oregano, 1/2 teaspoon garlic powder, and 1/4 teaspoon salt. Grill until everything is cooked through. Serve with 1/2 cup cooked quinoa and 1 cup roasted vegetables.

Day 12

· Breakfast:

Chia seed pudding. Mix 1/4 cup chia seeds, 1 cup unsweetened almond milk, 1 tablespoon honey, and 1/2 teaspoon vanilla extract. Refrigerate overnight. Top with fresh berries.

· Lunch:

Salmon Quinoa Bowl. Cook 1/2 cup quinoa according to package directions. Top with 4 ounces of grilled salmon, 1/4 cup sliced avocado, 1/4 cup sliced cucumber, and 1/4 cup sliced red onion. Coat with olive oil and lemon juice.

· Dinner:

Salmon and asparagus. Preheat oven to 400°F. Place 4 salmon fillets and 1 bunch of asparagus on a baking sheet. Coat with olive oil and sprinkle with salt and pepper. Bake for 12 to 15 minutes, until salmon is cooked through and asparagus is tender.

Day 13

· Breakfast:

 Mediterranean Breakfast Bowl. Follow the package instructions to cook 1/2 cup of quinoa. Top with 1/4 cup hummus, 1/4 cup chopped tomatoes, 1/4 cup chopped cucumber, 1/4 cup crumbled feta cheese, and 1/4 cup Kalamata olives.

· Lunch:

Mediterranean Tuna Salad. 1 can drained tuna, 1/4 cup chopped kalamata olives, 1/4 cup chopped red onion, 1/4 cup chopped cucumber, 1/4 cup chopped tomatoes, 1/4 cup crumbled feta cheese. Coat with olive oil and lemon juice.

· Dinner:

 Mediterranean grilled chicken. Season the chicken breast from step 4 with 1 teaspoon dried oregano, 1/2 teaspoon garlic powder, and 1/4 teaspoon salt. Grill until everything is cooked through. Serve with 1/2 cup cooked quinoa and 1 cup roasted vegetables.

Day 14

• Breakfast:

Greek yogurt parfait. Combine 1 cup plain Greek yogurt, 1/2 cup mixed berries, and 1/4 cup granola in a glass.

• Lunch:

Salmon Quinoa Bowl. Cook 1/2 cup quinoa according to package directions. Top with 4 ounces of grilled salmon, 1/4 cup sliced avocado, 1/4 cup sliced cucumber, and 1/4 cup sliced red onion. Coat with olive oil and lemon juice.

• Dinner:

Salmon and asparagus. Preheat oven to 400°F. Place 4 salmon fillets and 1 bunch of asparagus on a baking sheet. Coat with olive oil and sprinkle with salt and pepper. Bake for 12 to 15 minutes, until salmon is cooked through and asparagus is tender.

Day 15

• Breakfast:

Mediterranean Frittata. Whisk 4 eggs with 1/4 cup milk. Add 1/4 cup chopped tomatoes, 1/4 cup chopped spinach, 1/4 cup chopped mushrooms, and 1/4 cup crumbled feta cheese. Cook in a non-stick pot over medium heat until set.

• Lunch:

Mediterranean Wrap. Spread 2 tablespoons of hummus on whole wheat wrap. Top with 1/4 cup mixed vegetables, 1/4 cup chopped tomatoes, 1/4 cup chopped cucumber, 1/4 cup sliced red onion, 1/4 cup crumbled feta cheese, and 1/4 cup Kalamata olives. Roll it up and cut it in half.

• Dinner:

Mediterranean Stuffed Zucchini. Cut 4 zucchini in half lengthwise and scoop out the seeds. In a bowl, combine 1 pound ground turkey, 1/2 cup cooked quinoa, 1/4 cup chopped

Kalamata olives, 1/4 cup crumbled feta cheese, 1/4 cup chopped parsley, and 1/2 teaspoon dried oregano. Use 2 teaspoons of garlic powder and 1/4 teaspoon of salt. Stuff the zucchini with the turkey mixture. Bake at 180°C for 30-35 minutes, until the zucchini is soft and the inside is cooked through.

Day 16

• **Breakfast:**

Blueberry Almond Smoothie. Mix 1 cup unsweetened almond milk, 1/2 cup frozen blueberries, 1/2 banana, 1 tablespoon almond butter, and 1/2 teaspoon honey until smooth.

• **Lunch:**

Turkey Hummus Wrap. Spread 2 tablespoons of hummus on whole wheat wrap. Top with 2 turkey breast slices, 1/4 cup cucumber slices, 1/4 cup red onion slices, and 1/4 cup mixed vegetables. Roll it up and cut it in half.

• **Dinner:**

Mediterranean stuffed peppers with meat. Cut off the tops of 4 peppers and remove the seeds. In a bowl, combine 1 pound ground turkey, 1/2 cup cooked quinoa, 1/4 cup chopped Kalamata olives, 1/4 cup crumbled feta cheese, 1/4 cup chopped parsley, and 1/2 teaspoon dried oregano. Use 2 teaspoons of garlic powder and 1/4 teaspoon of salt. Stuff the peppers with the turkey mixture. Bake at 180C for 30-35 minutes, until the peppers are soft and the filling is cooked through.

Day 17

• **Breakfast:**

Mediterranean Breakfast Bowl. Follow the package instructions to cook 1/2 cup of quinoa. Top with 1/4 cup hummus, 1/4 cup chopped tomatoes, 1/4 cup chopped cucumber, 1/4 cup crumbled feta cheese, and 1/4 cup Kalamata olives.

• **Lunch:**

Mediterranean Tuna Salad. 1 can drained tuna, 1/4 cup chopped kalamata olives, 1/4 cup chopped red onion, 1/4 cup chopped cucumber, 1/4 cup chopped tomatoes, 1/4 cup crumbled feta cheese. Coat with olive oil and lemon juice.

• **Dinner:**

Mediterranean grilled chicken. Season the chicken breast from step 4 with 1 teaspoon dried oregano, 1/2 teaspoon garlic powder, and 1/4 teaspoon salt. Grill until everything is cooked through. Serve with 1/2 cup cooked quinoa and 1 cup roasted vegetables

Day 18

• **Breakfast:**

Chia Seed Pudding. Mix 1/4 cup chia seeds, 1 cup unsweetened almond milk, 1 tablespoon honey, and 1/2 teaspoon vanilla extract. Refrigerate overnight. Top with fresh berries.

• **Lunch:**

Salmon Quinoa Bowl. Follow the package instructions to cook 1/2 cup of quinoa. Top with 4 ounces of grilled salmon, 1/4 cup sliced avocado, 1/4 cup sliced cucumber, and 1/4 cup sliced red onion. Coat with olive oil and lemon juice.

• **Dinner:**

Salmon and asparagus. Preheat oven to 400°F. Place 4 salmon fillets and 1 bunch of asparagus on a baking sheet. Coat with olive oil and sprinkle with salt and pepper. Bake for 12 to 15 minutes, until salmon is cooked through and asparagus is tender.

Day 19

• **Breakfast:**

Greek yogurt parfait. Combine 1 cup plain Greek yogurt, 1/2 cup mixed berries, and 1/4 cup granola in a glass.

• **Lunch:**

Mediterranean Wrap. Spread 2 tablespoons of hummus on whole wheat wrap. Top with 1/4 cup mixed vegetables, 1/4 cup chopped tomatoes, 1/4 cup chopped cucumber, 1/4 cup sliced red onion, 1/4 cup crumbled feta cheese, and 1/4 cup Kalamata olives. Roll it up and cut it in half.

· Dinner:

Mediterranean Stuffed Zucchini. Cut 4 zucchini in half lengthwise and scoop out the seeds. In a bowl, combine 1 pound ground turkey, 1/2 cup cooked quinoa, 1/4 cup chopped Kalamata olives, 1/4 cup crumbled feta cheese, 1/4 cup chopped parsley, and 1/2 teaspoon dried oregano. Use 2 teaspoons of garlic powder and 1/4 teaspoon of salt. Stuff the zucchini with the turkey mixture. Bake at 180°C for 30-35 minutes, until the zucchini is soft and the inside is cooked through.

Day 20

· Breakfast:

 Mediterranean Frittata. Whisk 4 eggs with 1/4 cup milk. Add 1/4 cup chopped tomatoes, 1/4 cup chopped spinach, 1/4 cup chopped mushrooms, and 1/4 cup crumbled feta cheese. Cook in a non-stick pot over medium heat until set.

· Lunch:

Salmon Quinoa Bowl. Cook Follow the package instructions to cook 1/2 cup of quinoa. Top with 4 ounces of grilled salmon, 1/4 cup sliced avocado, 1/4 cup sliced cucumber, and 1/4 cup sliced red onion. Coat with olive oil and lemon juice.

· Dinner:

Salmon and asparagus. Preheat oven to 400°F. Place 4 salmon fillets and 1 bunch of asparagus on a baking sheet. Coat with olive oil and sprinkle with salt and pepper. Bake for 12 to 15 minutes, until salmon is cooked through and asparagus is tender.

Day 21

· Breakfast:

Blueberry Almond Smoothie. Mix 1 cup unsweetened almond milk, 1/2 cup frozen blueberries, 1/2 banana, 1 tablespoon almond butter, and 1/2 teaspoon honey until smooth.

· Lunch:

Mediterranean Tuna Salad. 1 can drained tuna, 1/4 cup chopped kalamata olives, 1/4 cup chopped red onion, 1/4 cup chopped cucumber, 1/4 cup chopped tomatoes, 1/4 cup crumbled feta cheese. Coat with olive oil and lemon juice.

· Dinner:

Mediterranean grilled chicken. Season the chicken breast from step 4 with 1 teaspoon dried oregano, 1/2 teaspoon garlic powder, and 1/4 teaspoon salt. Grill until everything is cooked through. Serve with 1/2 cup cooked quinoa and 1 cup roasted vegetables.

CHAPTER 5: DIETARY COMBINATIONS

The DASH, Mediterranean diet, and MIND diet are all healthy eating plans proven to improve overall health and reduce the risk of chronic disease. Combining these meals will give you the most health benefits.

The DASH diet emphasizes intake of fruits, vegetables, whole grains, lean proteins, and low-fat dairy while limiting intake of sodium, saturated fat, and added sugars.

The Mediterranean diet is rich in fruits, vegetables, whole grains, fish, and healthy fats such as olive oil, but limits red meat and processed foods.

The MIND diet is a combination of the DASH diet and the Mediterranean diet, which focuses on eating foods rich in nutrients such as vitamins, minerals, and antioxidants.

These foods include leafy greens, berries, nuts, whole grains, fish, and poultry.

This diet also recommends limiting your intake of unhealthy foods such as red meat, butter, cheese, and fried foods.

To combine these meals, you can start by incorporating more fruits, vegetables, whole grains, and lean protein into your diet while reducing your intake of sodium, saturated fat, and added sugars.

You can also replace unhealthy fats like butter and margarine with healthy fats like olive oil.

Additionally, you can eat more fish and poultry while limiting your intake of red meat and processed foods.

Finally, you can include more leafy greens, berries, and nuts in your diet to increase absorption of nutrients and antioxidants.

Recent studies have shown that combining the DASH, Mediterranean, and MIND diets provides the greatest health benefits.

A study published in the British Journal of Nutrition found that following a MIND-like diet significantly improved left ventricular function of the heart.

Another study found that combining DASH with a Mediterranean diet reduces the risk of cognitive decline and dementia2.

So it's worth considering incorporating these meals into your lifestyle to reap the benefits.

• **Tips for adhering to a combination diet**

Here are some tips for adhering to a combination diet:

1. **Focus on whole foods**: Fruits, vegetables, whole grains, low fat Include plenty of protein and healthy fats in your diet. These foods form the basis of the DASH, Mediterranean, and MIND diets and provide a wealth of nutrients and health benefits.

2. **Limit processed foods**: Processed foods are often high in sodium, sugar, and unhealthy fats, which can lead to a variety of health problems. Limit your intake of processed foods and choose whole foods instead.

3. **Choose healthy fats:** Healthy fats, such as those found in olive oil, nuts, and fatty fish, are an important part of the Mediterranean and MIND diets. These fats may help reduce inflammation, improve brain function, and reduce your risk of heart disease.

4. **Reduce Sodium Intake**: The DASH diet is designed to lower blood pressure, and one of the main ways it does this is by

reducing sodium intake. Try to limit your intake of foods high in sodium, such as processed meats, canned soups, and fast foods.

5. **Mindful Eating**: Mindful eating is an important part of the MIND diet and involves paying attention to your food and eating slowly without distractions. That way, you can enjoy your food more and eat less.

6. **Stay hydrated**: Drinking plenty of water is important for your overall health and helps you feel full and satisfied. Drink at least 8 cups of water per day.

7. **Get enough sleep**: Sleep is essential for good health, reducing stress, improving brain function, and reducing the risk of chronic disease. Sleep for 7 to 9 hours every night.

CHAPTER 6: EXERCISE AND HEALTHY AGING ABSOLUTELY

Exercise is an essential part of healthy aging. It helps maintain physical and mental health, improve quality of life, and reduce the risk of chronic disease.

This explains the importance of exercise for healthy aging and provides some tips for incorporating exercise into your daily life.

Exercise is essential to maintaining physical health as we age. It helps to maintain flexibility, balance, and coordination, which can also help prevent falls and other injuries. In addition to its physical benefits, exercise is also important for maintaining mental health as we age.

Exercise has been shown to reduce your risk of depression, anxiety, and cognitive decline, and improve our overall mood and sense of well-being. Exercise also helps maintain social connections. This is important for healthy aging.

There are many different types of exercise that can help you age healthily.

Aerobic exercise such as walking, running, and swimming can help improve cardiovascular health and reduce the risk of chronic diseases such as heart disease, stroke, and diabetes.

Strength training, such as weight lifting and resistance band exercises, can help maintain muscle mass and bone density, which are important for healthy aging.

Flexibility and balance exercises, such as yoga and tai chi, can help maintain mobility, balance, and coordination and prevent falls and other injuries.

It is important to note that you do not necessarily need to perform high-intensity exercise to reap the benefits of physical activity.

Even moderate physical activity, such as walking or gardening, can have positive effects on your health.

The key is to find activities that you enjoy and can do on a regular basis.

Here are some tips on how to incorporate exercise into your daily life.

1. **Start slow**. If you are new to exercise or have not exercised in a while, it is important to start slow and gradually increase your activity level. Start with low-intensity activities like walking or light stretching, and gradually increase the intensity and duration of your workouts.

2. **Find an activity you enjoy**: Exercise doesn't have to be a chore. Find an activity you enjoy, like dancing, swimming, or hiking, and make it a regular routine.

3. **Make it a habit**: The key to training is consistency. Make exercise a part of your daily routine, such as taking a walk after dinner or attending a yoga class every Saturday morning.

4. **Mix and match**: Incorporating different types of exercise into your daily routine can keep things interesting and prevent boredom. Keep your workouts fresh and exciting by trying different activities like swimming, cycling, and strength training.

5. **Socialize**: Exercising with others is a great way to stay motivated and make exercise more fun. Take a fitness class, a dance class, or find a workout girlfriend partner to keep you accountable.

6. **Listen to your body**: It's important to listen to your body and avoid over exercising. If you experience pain or discomfort while exercising, slow or stop your movements and consult your doctor.

In summary, exercise is an essential part of healthy aging.

Regular exercise helps maintain physical and mental health, improves quality of life, and reduces the risk of chronic disease. Incorporating exercise into your daily life and following these tips will help you stay healthy and active as you age.

• Tips for staying active as you get older absolutely

Staying active as you age is important for maintaining your physical and mental health, improving your quality of life, and reducing your risk of chronic disease.

Here are some tips to stay active as you get older:

1. **Participate in aerobic exercise**: Aerobic exercise, such as brisk walking, jogging, cycling, swimming, and aerobics classes, helps keep you active as you age. Layering is an important part of staying active. Aim to do at least 30 minutes of aerobic exercise per day, 5 days per week.

2. **Incorporate strength training**: Strength training, such as weight lifting and resistance band exercises, can help maintain muscle mass and bone density, which are important for healthy aging. Try to participate in strength training at least two days a week.

3. **Incorporate flexibility and balance exercises**: Flexibility and balance exercises, such as yoga and tai chi, can help maintain mobility, balance, and coordination and prevent falls and other injuries. Participate in flexibility and balance exercises at least two days a week.

4. **Stay active throughout the day**: In addition to structured training, it is important to stay active throughout the day. Take the stairs instead of the elevator, walk to the store instead of the car, or take a walk during your lunch break.

5. **Find an activity you enjoy**: Exercise doesn't have to be a chore. Find an activity you enjoy, like dancing, swimming, or hiking, and make it a regular routine.

6. **Make it social**: Exercising with others is a great way to stay motivated and make exercise more fun. Take fitness or dance class, or find a workout partner to keep you accountable.

7. **Listen to your body**: It's important to listen to your body and avoid over exercising. If you experience pain or discomfort while exercising, slow or stop your movements and consult your doctor.

8. **Stay hydrated**: Drinking plenty of water is important for your overall health and helps you feel full and satisfied. Drink at least 8 cups of water per day.

9. **Get enough sleep**: Sleep is essential for good health, reducing stress, improving brain function, and reducing the risk of chronic disease. Sleep for 7 to 9 hours every night.

10. **Healthy Eating**: A healthy diet is important for staying active as you age.

Aim for a diet rich in fruits, vegetables, whole grains, lean protein, and healthy fats.

CHAPTER 7: MENTAL HEALTH AND HEALTHY AGING

As we age, we may experience a variety of physical and emotional changes that can affect our mental health.

These changes may include chronic health conditions, cognitive decline, social isolation, and loss of loved ones.

This explains the importance of mental health for healthy aging and provides some tips for maintaining good mental health as you age.

Mental health is important for maintaining overall health as we age. Good mental health allows you to maintain relationships, stay engaged with your community, and enjoy hobbies and interests.

Mental health not only impacts your overall well-being but is also important for maintaining physical health as you age.

Poor mental health not only increases the risk of chronic diseases such as heart disease, stroke, and diabetes, but also affects the immune system and increases the risk of infections.

A variety of factors can affect your mental health as you grow older.

These include chronic health conditions, cognitive decline, social isolation, and loss of loved ones.

It is important to be aware of these risk factors and take steps to eliminate them.

In summary, mental health is an essential part of healthy aging.

Good mental health helps maintain overall health, cope with the challenges of aging, and reduce the risk of chronic disease.

• Tips for maintaining good mental health as you age

Here are some tips for maintaining good mental health as you age.

1. **Stay connected**: Maintaining social connections is important for mental health. Stay in touch with friends and family, join a club or organization, or volunteer in your community.

2. **Stay active**: Regular exercise is important for maintaining good mental health. Exercise can help reduce stress, improve your mood, and improve your overall health.

3. **Healthy Eating**: Healthy eating is important for maintaining good mental health. Maintain a diet rich in fruits, vegetables, whole grains, lean proteins, and healthy fats.

4. **Get enough sleep**: Sleep is essential for mental health. Sleep for 7 to 9 hours every night.

5. **Managing stress**: Stress can affect your mental health and increase your risk of chronic disease. Find healthy ways to deal with stress, such as meditation, yoga, and breathing exercises.

6. **Ask for help if you need it**: If you are struggling with your mental health, don't hesitate to ask for help. Talk to your doctor, mental health professional or trusted friend or family member.

CHAPTER 8: CONCLUSION KEY POINTS FROM THE BOOK

Discover the secret to a long, vibrant life and revitalize your health with the DASH, Mediterranean, and MIND diets: The ultimate guide to healthy aging.

The key points are:

1. The DASH, Mediterranean, and MIND diets are all effective for healthy aging. These diets emphasize whole foods, lean proteins, healthy fats, and lots of fruits and vegetables.

2. Exercise is an essential part of healthy aging. Regular exercise helps maintain physical and mental health, improves quality of life, and reduces the risk of chronic disease.

3. Mental health is important for maintaining overall health as we age. Good mental health allows you to maintain relationships, stay engaged with your community, and enjoy hobbies and interests.

4. Social contact is important for mental health. Stay in touch with friends and family, join a club or organization, or volunteer in your community.

5. Stress management is important for mental health. Find healthy ways to deal with stress, such as meditation, yoga, and

breathing exercises.

6. Sleep is essential for mental health. Sleep for 7 to 9 hours every night.

7. A healthy diet is important for maintaining physical and mental health. Maintain a diet rich in fruits, vegetables, whole grains, lean proteins, and healthy fats.

8. Stay active throughout the day. In addition to structured training, it is important to stay active throughout the day. Take the stairs instead of the elevator, walk to the store instead of the car, or take a walk during your lunch break.

9. Listen to your body. It's important to listen to your body and avoid over exercising. If you experience pain or discomfort while exercising, slow or stop your movements and consult your doctor.

10. Drink enough. Drinking plenty of water is important for your overall health and helps you feel full and satisfied. Drink at least 8 cups of water per day.

By following these key insights, you can create a healthy, balanced lifestyle that incorporates the best aspects of the DASH, Mediterranean, and MIND diets.

• Final Thoughts on Healthy Aging In summary, healthy aging is a multifaceted process that involves managing physical, mental, and emotional health.

By following the tips outlined in this conversation, you can create a healthy, balanced lifestyle that incorporates the best of the DASH, Mediterranean, and MIND diets.

Focus on whole foods, stay active, maintain mental health, stay connected to others, manage stress, get enough sleep, eat healthy, and stay active throughout the day.

Don't forget to spend time. Listen to your body and drink plenty of water.

By keeping these tips in mind, you can improve your overall health and well-being and reduce your risk of chronic disease.

It's important to remember that healthy aging is a journey, not a destination. It's never too late to take care of your health and make positive changes in your life. By taking small steps every day, you can improve your health and well-being and enjoy a long, fulfilling life.

Combined recipes from the DASH, Mediterranean, and MIND diets:

1. **Mediterranean Quinoa Salad**: This salad is packed with nutrients and antioxidants. It contains quinoa, which is a great source of protein and fiber, as well as fresh herbs and vegetables that are rich in nutrients and antioxidants. The dressing is made from olive oil, a healthy fat that is a staple of the Mediterranean diet. This salad is also free of sodium, an important component of the DASH diet

2. **Mediterranean Chicken**: This dish is a great source of lean protein and healthy fats. It contains chicken, which is a good source of protein, and is flavored with antioxidant-rich herbs and spices. This dish is also served with roasted vegetables, which are a good source of fiber and nutrients.

3. **Mediterranean Fish**: This dish is an excellent source of omega-3 fatty acids, which are essential for brain health. It contains fish, a good source of protein and omega-3 fatty acids, and is flavored with antioxidant-rich herbs and spices. This dish is also served with roasted vegetables, which are a good source of fiber and nutrients.

4. **Mediterranean Lentil Soup**: This soup is a good source of protein and fiber. Contains lentils, which are a good source of protein and fiber, and fresh herbs and vegetables, which are rich in nutrients and antioxidants. The soup also has no salt, which is an important part of the DASH diet.

5. **Mediterranean Stuffed Peppers**: This dish is a great source of

fiber and nutrients. These include bell peppers, which are a good source of fiber and nutrients, and lean ground turkey, which is a good source of protein. This dish is flavored with antioxidant-rich herbs and spices.

6. Mediterranean Chicken Skewers: This dish is a great source of lean protein and healthy fats. It contains chicken, which is a good source of protein, and is flavored with antioxidant-rich herbs and spices. This dish is also served with roasted vegetables, which are a good source of fiber and nutrients.

7. Mediterranean Tuna Salad: This salad is packed with nutrients and antioxidants. It contains tuna, which is an excellent source of protein and omega-3 fatty acids, as well as fresh herbs and vegetables rich in nutrients and antioxidants. The dressing is made from olive oil, a healthy fat that is a staple of the Mediterranean diet. This salad is also low in sodium, which is an important part of the DASH diet.

8. Mediterranean Stuffed Zucchini: This dish is a great source of fiber and nutrients. Contains zucchini, a good source of fiber and nutrients, and lean ground turkey, and a good source of protein.

This dish is flavored with antioxidant-rich herbs and spices.

9. Mediterranean Quinoa Bowl: This bowl is packed with nutrients and antioxidants. It contains quinoa, which is a great source of protein and fiber, as well as fresh herbs and vegetables that are rich in nutrients and antioxidants. The bowl is also topped with a poached egg, which is a great source of protein.

10. Mediterranean Baked Salmon: This dish is an excellent source of omega-3 fatty acids, which are essential for brain health. It contains salmon, a good source of protein and omega-3 fatty acids, and is flavored with antioxidant-rich herbs and spices. This dish is also served with roasted vegetables, which are a good source of fiber and nutrients.

11. **Stuffed Mediterranean Peppers**: This dish is a great source of fiber and nutrients. These include bell peppers, which are a good source of fiber and nutrients, and lean ground turkey, which is a good source of protein. This dish is flavored with antioxidant-rich herbs and spices.

12. **Mediterranean Chicken**: This dish is a great source of lean protein and healthy fats. It contains chicken, which is a good source of protein, and is flavored with antioxidant-rich herbs and spices. This dish is also served with roasted vegetables, which are a good source of fiber and nutrients.

13. **Mediterranean Fish**: This dish is an excellent source of omega-3 fatty acids, which are essential for brain health. It contains fish, a good source of protein and omega-3 fatty acids, and is flavored with antioxidant-rich herbs and spices. This dish is also served with roasted vegetables, which are a good source of fiber and nutrients.

14. **Mediterranean Quinoa Salad**: This salad is packed with nutrients and antioxidants. It contains quinoa, which is a great source of protein and fiber, as well as fresh herbs and vegetables that are rich in nutrients and antioxidants. The dressing is made from olive oil, a healthy fat that is a staple of the Mediterranean diet. This salad is also low in sodium, which is an important part of the DASH diet.

15. **Mediterranean Chicken Skewers**: This dish is a great source of lean protein and healthy fats. It contains chicken, which is a good source of protein, and is flavored with antioxidant-rich herbs and spices. This dish is also served with roasted vegetables, which are a good source of fiber and nutrients.

16. **Mediterranean Tuna Salad**: This salad is packed with nutrients and antioxidants. It contains tuna, which is an excellent source of protein and omega-3 fatty acids, as well as fresh herbs and vegetables rich in nutrients and antioxidants. The dressing is made from olive oil, a healthy fat that is a staple of the Mediterranean diet. This salad is also low in sodium, which is an

important part of the DASH diet.

17. **Mediterranean Stuffed Zucchini**: This dish is a great source of fiber and nutrients. Contains zucchini, a good source of fiber and nutrients, and lean ground turkey, and a good source of protein. This dish is flavored with antioxidant-rich herbs and spices.

18. **Mediterranean Quinoa Bowl:** This bowl is packed with nutrients and antioxidants. It contains quinoa, which is a great source of protein and fiber, as well as fresh herbs and vegetables that are rich in nutrients and antioxidants. The bowl is also topped with a poached egg, which is a great source of protein.

19. **Mediterranean Baked Salmon**: This dish is an excellent source of omega-3 fatty acids, which are essential for brain health. It contains salmon, a good source of protein and omega-3 fatty acids, and is flavored with antioxidant-rich herbs and spices. This dish is also served with roasted vegetables, which are a good source of fiber and nutrients.

20. **Mediterranean Lentil Soup**: This soup is a good source of protein and fiber. Contains lentils, which are a good source of protein and fiber, and fresh herbs and vegetables, which are rich in nutrients and antioxidants. The soup also has no salt, which is an important part of the DASH diet.

How do I make these recipes?

Here are the steps to prepare the above recipes.

1. **Mediterranean Quinoa Salad**: Wash quinoa through a fine sieve and drain. Start by boiling quinoa and water in a medium saucepan. Reduce heat and simmer for 15 to 20 minutes or until quinoa is tender and liquid is absorbed. In a small bowl, combine olive oil, lemon juice, honey, salt, and black pepper. In a large bowl, combine cooked quinoa, parsley, mint, basil, cucumber, cherry tomatoes, and red onion. Pour dressing over salad and mix. Top with crumbled feta cheese and chopped walnuts.

2. **Mediterranean Chicken**: Preheat oven to 375°F. Season the

chicken breasts with salt, pepper, and dried oregano. Warm the olive oil in a large skillet that can be placed in the oven, over medium heat. Add the chicken breasts and fry until golden brown, 2 to 3 minutes on each side. Place the pan in the oven and bake for 15-20 minutes or until the chicken is cooked through. Serve with roasted vegetables.

3. **Mediterranean Fish**: Preheat oven to 400°F. Season the fish fillets with salt, pepper, and dried oregano. Warm the olive oil in a large skillet that can be placed in the oven, over medium heat. Add the fish fillets and fry until golden brown, 2 to 3 minutes on each side. Place the pan in the oven and bake for 10-12 minutes or until the fish is cooked through. Serve with roasted vegetables.

4. **Mediterranean Lentil Soup**: Warm the olive oil in a large skillet that can be placed in the oven, over medium heat. Add onions, carrots, and celery and cook for 5 to 7 minutes or until vegetables are tender. Add garlic and cook for another minute. Add the lentils, chicken stock, diced tomatoes, oregano, and bay leaf. Bring the soup to a boil, then reduce the heat and simmer for 30-40 minutes, or until the lentils are tender. Remove the bay leaf and add salt and black pepper to the soup.

5. **Mediterranean Stuffed Peppers**: Preheat oven to 375°F. Take off the tops of the peppers and get rid of the seeds. In a large bowl, combine ground turkey, cooked quinoa, cherry tomatoes, red onion, garlic, oregano, salt, and black pepper. Stuff the peppers with the mixture and place in a baking dish. Bake for 25-30 minutes or until the peppers are soft and the filling is cooked through.

6. **Mediterranean Chicken Skewers**: Preheat grill to medium-high heat. In a small bowl, combine olive oil, lemon juice, garlic, oregano, salt, and black pepper. Thread the chicken onto skewers and brush with the marinade. Grill chicken skewers for 10-12 minutes or until cooked through. Serve with tzatziki sauce.

7. **Mediterranean Tuna Salad**: In a large bowl, combine tuna, cucumber, cherry tomatoes, red onion, olives, and feta cheese. In

a small bowl, combine olive oil, lemon juice, garlic, oregano, salt, and black pepper. Pour dressing over salad and mix.

8. **Mediterranean Stuffed Zucchini:** Preheat oven to 375°F. Slice the zucchini in half lengthwise and scoop out the seeds. In a large bowl, combine ground turkey, cooked quinoa, cherry tomatoes, red onion, garlic, oregano, salt, and black pepper. Pour the mixture over the zucchini halves and place in a baking dish. Bake for 25-30 minutes or until zucchini is tender and stuffing is cooked through.

9. **Mediterranean Quinoa Bowl**: Wash quinoa through a fine sieve and drain. Start by boiling quinoa and water in a medium saucepan. Reduce heat and simmer for 15 to 20 minutes or until quinoa is tender and liquid is absorbed. In a small bowl, combine olive oil, lemon juice, garlic, oregano, salt, and black pepper. In a large bowl, combine cooked quinoa, chickpeas, cucumber, cherry tomatoes, red onion, and feta cheese. Pour the dressing into a bowl and stir to combine.

10. **Baked Mediterranean Salmon**: Preheat oven to 400°F. Season the salmon fillets with salt, pepper, and dried oregano. Warm the olive oil in a large skillet that can be placed in the oven, over medium heat. Add the salmon fillets and fry for 2-3 minutes on each side until golden brown. Place the skillet in the oven and bake for 10-12 minutes or until the salmon is cooked through. Serve with roasted vegetables.

11. **Mediterranean Stuffed Peppers**: Preheat oven to 375°F. Take off the tops of the peppers and get rid of the seeds. In a large bowl, combine ground turkey, cooked quinoa, cherry tomatoes, red onion, garlic, oregano, salt, and black pepper. Fill the peppers with the mixture and put them in a baking dish. Bake for 25-30 minutes or until the peppers are soft and the filling is cooked through.

12. **Mediterranean Chicken**: Preheat oven to 375°F. Season the chicken breasts with salt, pepper, and dried oregano. Warm the olive oil in a large skillet that can be placed in the oven, over medium heat. Add the chicken breasts and fry until golden brown,

2 to 3 minutes on each side. Place the pan in the oven and bake for 15-20 minutes or until the chicken is cooked through. Serve with roasted vegetables.

14. **Mediterranean Fish:** Preheat oven to 400°F. Season the fish fillets with salt, pepper, and dried oregano. Warm the olive oil in a large skillet that can be placed in the oven, over medium heat. Add the fish fillets and fry until golden brown, 2 to 3 minutes on each side. Place the pan in the oven and bake for 10-12 minutes or until the fish is cooked through. Serve with roasted vegetables.

15. **Mediterranean Quinoa Salad**: Rinse the quinoa in a fine-mesh colander and drain. Start by boiling quinoa and water in a medium saucepan. Reduce heat and simmer for 15 to 20 minutes or until quinoa is tender and liquid is absorbed. In a small bowl, combine olive oil, lemon juice, honey, salt, and black pepper. In a large bowl, combine cooked quinoa, parsley, mint, basil, cucumber, cherry tomatoes, and red onion. Pour dressing over salad and mix. Sprinkle crumbled feta cheese and chopped walnuts on top.

16. **Mediterranean Chicken Skewers:** Preheat grill to medium-high heat. In a small bowl, combine olive oil, lemon juice, garlic, oregano, salt, and black pepper. Thread the chicken onto skewers and brush with the marinade. Grill chicken skewers for 10-12 minutes or until cooked through. Serve with tzatziki sauce.

17. **Mediterranean Tuna Salad:** In a large bowl, combine the tuna, cucumber, cherry tomatoes, red onion, olives, and feta cheese. In a small bowl, combine olive oil, lemon juice, garlic, oregano, salt, and black pepper. Pour dressing over salad and mix.

18. **Mediterranean Stuffed Zucchini**: Preheat oven to 375°F. Slice the zucchini in half lengthwise and scoop out the seeds. In a large bowl, combine ground turkey, cooked quinoa, cherry tomatoes, red onion, garlic, oregano, salt, and black pepper. Pour the mixture over the zucchini halves and place in a baking dish. Bake for 25-30 minutes or until zucchini is tender and stuffing is cooked through.

19. **Mediterranean Quinoa Bowl**: Wash quinoa through a fine sieve and drain. Start by boiling quinoa and water in a medium saucepan. Reduce heat and simmer for 15 to 20 minutes or until quinoa is tender and liquid is absorbed. In a small bowl, combine olive oil, lemon juice, garlic, oregano, salt, and black pepper. In a large bowl, combine cooked quinoa, chickpeas, cucumber, cherry tomatoes, red onion, and feta cheese. Pour the dressing into a bowl and stir to combine.

20. **Mediterranean Baked Salmon**: Preheat oven to 400°F. Season the salmon fillets with salt, pepper, and dried oregano. Warm the olive oil in a large skillet that can be placed in the oven, over medium heat. Add the salmon fillets and fry for 2-3 minutes on each side until golden brown. Place the skillet in the oven and bake for 10-12 minutes or until the salmon is cooked through. Serve with roasted vegetables.

21. **Mediterranean Lentil Soup**: Heat the olive oil in a large pot over medium heat. Add onions, carrots, and celery and cook for 5 to 7 minutes or until vegetables are tender. Add garlic and cook for another minute. Add the lentils, chicken stock, diced tomatoes, oregano, and bay leaf. Bring the soup to a boil, then reduce the heat and simmer for 30-40 minutes, or until the lentils are tender. Remove the bay leaf and add salt and black pepper to the soup.